A day of rest

So I am not put to the test

Of a poem to you

Who I love so true

But when Monday comes

And I hope with the sun

I will write my love in volumes

One by one.

Breakfast Memories

A Dementia Love Story

KATE HANLEY

Printed in the United States

10 9 8 7 6 5 4 3 2 1

Green Writers Press is a Vermont-based publisher whose mission is to spread a message of hope and renewal through the words and images we publish. We will adhere to our commitment to preserving and protecting the natural resources of the earth. To that end, a percentage of our proceeds will be donated to social-justice and environmental activist groups. Green Writers Press gratefully acknowledges the generosity of individual donors, friends, and readers to help support the environment and our publishing initiative. For information about funding or getting involved in our publishing program, contact Green Writers Press.

Giving Voice to Writers & Artists Who Will Make the World a Better Place
Green Writers Press | Brattleboro, Vermont
greenwriterspress.com

ISBN: 978-1-9505841-6-1 (paperback)
Memoir

First Edition

Printed by Cathedral Corporation
Design by Sarah Clarehart

DEDICATION
....

Dedicated to Manny & Marshal... Never forget that your first breaths will be remembered deep in my soul, when I take my last.

FOREWORD

....

Poetry inked on napkins, one of many that he left beside the breakfast he made for her daily, his last line of defense against the rising darkness of her dementia. The napkin, and dozens of others, just like it, each one covered in the outpourings of a man's heart.

HOLD ME
HOLD ME TIGHT
IN THE COMFORT OF THE DARKNESS
LET ME FEEL
YOUR SOFTNESS
YOUR STRENGTH AND SPIRIT
AN DREAM
OF WHAT CAN BE
SO I SHALL NOT FEAR

THE LIGHT OF REALITY

This is a story of love, and a love story. A story of what I saw and felt as a daughter when my mom experienced dementia, and how my father's love through their 65 years of marriage and courtship proved the definitive weapon against this disease.

This is a story of hope for all who are watching those they love lose their memories. It is my personal journey of how I learned that when one is stricken by dementia, the mind and memories are lost and forgotten. However, I witnessed, through the love of my father for my mother, that this disease does not hold power over the memories *that are stored within our souls.*

If you are the caregiver for one who has succumbed to the disease of dementia, please do not despair. You are doing the right thing. Your love and kindness will be remembered.

I've walked this path, and I know this.

CHAPTER 1

The Beauty Parlor Day

The newly laid mulch held a fresh scent and looked perfect with the array of promised daffodils popping through the ground from the April showers. In front of the basketball hoop, the chalk marks on the driveway outlining the boundaries for three-point shots were slightly washed away, faded from the spring rain. It was such a pretty day as we sat in the car in front of our home entrance and waited for her.

What was taking so long? Dad and Marshal were in the car ready to head to the toy shop for his birthday present.

"Bernadette," he yelled out to her from the car window. "Bernadette, we're waiting for you in the car."

She casually appeared at the doorway wearing the same red sweater from the day before, unflustered by his beckoning call. "Here I am," she said, with the smile that could light up a galaxy.

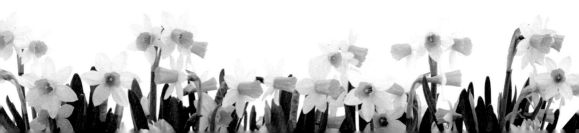

As Marsh got out and helped her into the front passenger seat, my insides tingled and I smiled, knowing just how much it meant to him to be with his grandparents. My husband and I both treasured these precious weekends when my parents would travel the two hours on the New York State Thruway and spend time with our two sons. Today was even more special as Dad and Marsh were going to shop for his ten-year-old's birthday present. The toy shop, located just four doors down in the same plaza as the beauty parlor where I had gifted Mom with a cut, color and style, was sure to have the newest Star Wars light saber. I was sure it was going to be another great weekend with my mom and dad.

I dropped off Mom first, at the sidewalk entrance of the salon. "Just call me when you're done," I said and kissed her cheek as I reached over to open her passenger door. "They've already been paid, so don't even think of trying to pay for this!" She giggled at my comment, as Dad added, "Don't change it too much!" It was no secret that he loved her auburn hair that held just a slight flip of a curl as it touched her slender shoulders. It would take quite the hairdresser to convince him that his wife of almost 55 years could look any prettier with a different-styled cut.

A few minutes later, I dropped off Marsh and Dad at the entrance to the toy store.

"We'll call you when we're done; give us an hour or so."

Perfect, I thought, knowing I would be back at that same time to pick up Mom. *Just enough time to get home, marinade the lamb chops for dinner, and make Marshal's birthday cake.*

The smell of fresh rosemary was finding its way from the cutting board to the chops, when my cell phone rang. I glanced at my phone and saw "Dad" on the screen.

Already? It had only been thirty minutes.

A quick flutter of anxiety shot through me as I grabbed a towel to wipe my hands from the garlic press to answer the call. "Dad, you OK?"

"Please come get us now," his voice pleading with a sense of despair. "Marsh and I just found your mother walking around the plaza. She never went into the salon. She said she forgot why she was here. Please come get us."

"Something is wrong with your mother."

I slid the roasting pan toward the back of the counter, turned off the oven, grabbed the keys, and did exactly what he asked.

The red traffic lights couldn't turn green fast enough. *I hope she is OK,* I thought as the sound of Dad's nervous voice from his call to me last month echoed in my mind with his concern that "something is wrong with your mother."

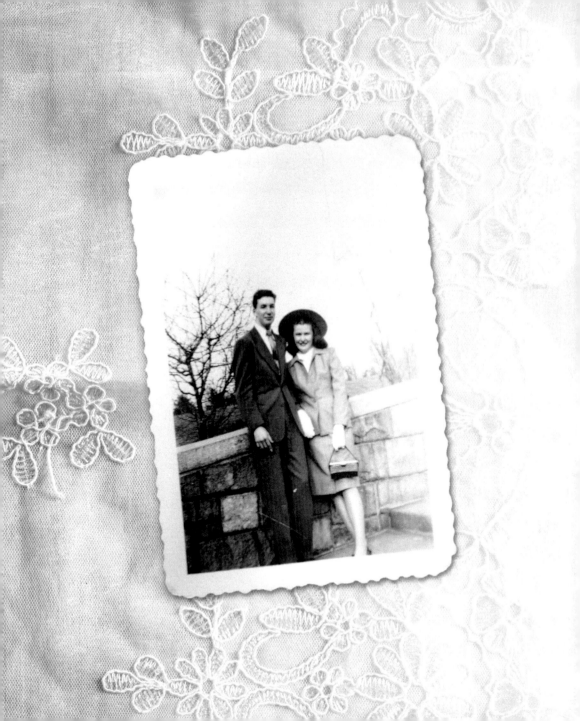

CHAPTER 2
....

Them

While we are growing up and caught up in childish and adolescent things, our parents' private lives are something of a mystery. It's even more complicated when it comes to who they were before we came along. We weren't there to witness events or register impressions, either behind the curtain of their privacy or their past.

What we're left to handle, when we try to reach for who they really are, are just the surface facts: our mundane daily encounters with them, some old photos, and a few wry or cute or terrible stories.

There comes a time when some of us feel compelled to excavate down through the layers, and think about who these people really were. One such time occurs when you start to lose them.

Then you dig, not so much with your mind, for bare facts—those are glaring. You dig with your heart. Like an archaeologist, you may only be left to guess at the meaning and purpose of what you uncover. But to do that is important—at least to the heart.

It was for mine.

"Hello, Miss O'Rourke. "

"Hello, Mr. McDonough."

That was their daily exchange as he picked her up from her job at B. Altman's, "America's Most Famous Department Store" on 5th and 34th Street in Midtown Manhattan.

She would come down the escalator, beaming from the top step with a ray of light that seemed to surround her, and gently wave at him in recognition, smiling shyly until she reached the main floor. She was always smiling. A smile with a humbleness that was ever enchanting as its warmth swept onto the avenues where they would walk out the department store entrance, stroll hand in hand, and chat.

1944

They met through her older brother, John. John and Dad both attended Manhattan's Saint Vincent Ferrer Catholic School and had mutual future plans to enlist in the Navy.

"Would it be OK if my little sister Bernadette joined us today for an ice cream soda?" John asked Dad one day after school, knowing full well that his little sister, the youngest of four in the O'Rourke family, with roots in County Leitrim, Ireland, might well steal Peter's heart. "She has a weakness for ice cream, and I think she'd enjoy your company."

And the rest, as they say, is history. John had been right. That was the day Peter saw her, and, as was his determined nature, knew he wanted to win her and keep her in his life. She was lovely, with big, sparkling blue eyes, and a terrific figure. She was sweetly shy yet engaging; she was brilliant yet humble and pure.

John went back to his studies, and Peter walked Bernadette back to her parents' home. He asked if she would join him the next day for a piece of chocolate cake. She said yes. They ended up instead at a 5th Avenue ice cream shop. It became their bond, meeting for ice cream after he picked her up from B. Altman's. She was so smart. She was going to apply to Hunter College after high school to study home economics. She was proud of herself, and oh so sweet, like the ice cream they would order on their dates.

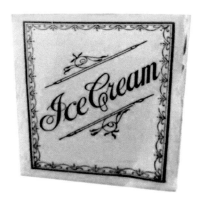

Ice cream box from their dating days

They shared stories of their childhoods, both having parents who left Ireland and immigrated to America with nothing but the clothes on their backs and the hope of finding love and building future generations. Mom's father was an ice delivery man and her mom was a housekeeper. Between the two incomes, there was enough money to cover the expenses of their small, three-room apartment in Manhattan. Bernadette was adored as a child by both of her parents and her siblings. She grew up expecting little, demanding nothing, and poured much into making her parents proud. Their house was filled with love and happy times that included college graduation celebrations of all four O'Rourke children—three of them women.

Dad's life was different economically, but similar in the virtue of family loyalty and pride. He grew up broke—the kind of broke illustrated in poverty scenes by Norman Rockwell. Unlike Mom, he didn't know his father well. His only memories were of his father in the hospital and his grisly, eventual death from lung disease due to mustard-gas poisoning during World War I. His mom, Bridget, and he were very close. She adored him, and he often accompanied her on her job as an office cleaner in old East-side Manhattan tenement buildings. When Dad wasn't working with Bridget or studying for school, he was responsible for smashing discarded crates on the street to provide firewood for heating their small-three room, fifth-floor apartment. Unlike Mom, Dad had no electricity as a child. No wood meant no heat for the family.

They dated for two years, and then Dad and her brother, John, went off to the Navy. Although John was the required enlistment age of eighteen, Dad was only seventeen. With fierce determination and loyalty to his mom, he graduated one year early from high school and, so that he could enter the military, falsified his date of birth and added one year to his age. Moreover, he changed his middle name on his military enlistment papers. In the 1940's the federal government offered veterans benefits for mothers of sons in the military. As a son devoted to the care of his mom, he entered the Navy with the faith and peace that she would be protected by the G.I. Bill should anything happen to him.

1945

He was stationed at Sampson Naval Base in Upstate New York where he wrote in the evenings to his girlfriend Bernadette. He wrote to her of his plans to return to Manhattan to see her, and…would she be waiting for him?

He wrote that he was interested in her thoughts on politics, her quiet but strong opinion, and the cheerful spirit that she carried in her personality. He wrote that the electric alarm clock in his room was wonderful and that his nights were filled with entertaining radio broadcasts from the common area of the compound main building. He gave her details of his day, hoping her mind would escape into his world and that she would miss him. He wrote of hoping her parents liked and respected him, his unspoken intention being that once he was out of the Navy, if she obliged, she would honor him and accept his marriage proposal.

1951

He was 23, a college graduate, and out of the Navy. She was 21, and had just graduated with honors from Hunter College three months earlier. They were married at the parish church she had attended her whole life. They had plans, big plans—plans to make a better world. Plans to make her parents and his mom feel a pride that only immigrants to America must feel as they watch their children—the family's first generation of Americans—flourish.

October 28, 1946: Peter's letter from Sampson Naval Base

Oct. 28, 7 PM

My dearest Bernadette
Today was a wonderful day, your letter made it so When I close the door of my room and sit down to read your letter all noise and everything fades away. It's just like I was home again talking to you. After reading your letter I want to jump on the first bus that will take me to you. I realize more each day that without you nothing would seem interesting. You understand all the things I say and do. Most of all I hope you understand I love you very much.
Your letter stated thirty one days.
give this it will be twenty six
are together again. You'll
I am to be coming
that day of the

TO: MISS BERNADETTE O'ROURKE

1953

As newlyweds, they had a small one-room apartment in Brooklyn. Their first-born, traditionally and lovingly named after Mom in the Irish Catholic practice, was born two years after their wedding. The baby thrived in their small apartment, partitioned by a curtain that created a makeshift nursery and held the small bassinet Peter built for his beautiful daughter. She was baptized within two days by the same priest who married them.

Two years later, Mary Margaret was born, named after Mom's two sisters. They moved to a bigger apartment in the same building, which included a real second room as a nursery for both girls.

"Bernadette, it's time to leave Brooklyn," he told her. "We need a better place to raise the girls."

Two years later, their first born son and Dad's namesake, was born in Philadelphia. I came along two years later and was named Catherine, after Mom's mother. I cannot imagine how anxious and exhausted she must have been with four little children, (one every two years,) a husband who earned his living as a traveling salesman, and her closest family support now four hours away in Manhattan. But overwhelming was not in her vocabulary and not a part of her being. Not our Mom, the home economist. She had a system.

She put her home economics degree to work by starting a shared babysitting business so that she and Dad could have one night a week without kids. Our CEO mother designed a business plan in Darby, outside of Philadelphia, where her neighbors and friends would watch her four toddlers for one night a week in exchange for her watching another family's children for the same amount of time. Brilliant economics, if you ask me. They had no money for babysitters; who would? They were raising four children on his one salary, but he would tell her not to worry about their financial future. Any good economist knows the future is all about worry, so sure enough, she took her love for being alone with her husband one night a week into her own hands without tendering cash. She kept her role as mother and as wife, as only she could have done. What a clever woman, yet again, creating and finding time to share her love and affection for our dad.

Two years later James, a.k.a. Jamesy, was born and named after Mom's uncle in Ireland. Dad had taken a better job making more money and was able to get a bigger house to provide for his wife and small little children, now five in tow, in their new home of Cincinnati, Ohio.

Two years later they moved to another suburb in Cincinnati, with a stronger Catholic elementary school in walking distance for my older siblings. Their sixth child, Thomas, my second youngest brother, came along and was christened and named after her sister Catherine's husband.

Two years later, my little sister Patricia, their seventh and final child, was born. Their last relocation, to a suburb in Rochester, New York, offered their brood of seven children a four-bedroom, one-bathroom, 1830 farmhouse. The house was set in a perfect village suburb with sidewalks everywhere and a short walk to the Catholic convent, where we attended religious education classes. The elementary school was literally in the backyard, and the middle school and high school were both a quick walk down the hill. This was really when my memories of childhood started, with the birth and naming of my sister Trish.

All six of us had been namesakes, but for some reason, naming this seventh child was different. She was not to be a namesake. This time, the six of us participated in the naming of our newborn sister.

"You have a little sister," Dad announced as he walked through the kitchen door, returning from the hospital. "The baby and your mother should be home in five days or so. We can go and see them both tomorrow. Your mother wants to name the baby Agnes."

"What? Agnes?" The scream from my older siblings and I could be heard throughout the neighborhood and the dinner table quickly turned into a competition on naming the baby, all of us, shouting out names for our little sister like we were on *Family Feud*. Poor little baby had no idea what world she was about to enter with such competitive brothers and sisters, each insisting that the name they had selected for the baby was the best. In the end, Dad claimed victory in the name game, after naming his lovely little baby girl after a beautiful girl he remembered from his elementary school youth. His victory was challenged by Mom, of course, who said the baby was named after two of her favorite saints.

For 45 years our family lived in the same house, hosted graduation parties for all seven of us from high school, pushed seven of us out the door to college and welcomed thirteen grandchildren. Our home was known throughout the village as "the Mayor's House," and Mom was "the Mayor's Wife," or as Bette Midler so beautifully sings, the "wind beneath [his] wings." To me, my brothers, and my sisters, she was simply a vessel of happy energy and unending love and faith.

Mom had a skip in her step, a smile that had the sweetness of the nectar that we read about in the story of Adam and Eve, and the work ethics of her beloved parents. Constantly using her home economics degree, she ran our home like a machine on all four gears. She had seven children—seven workers who helped manage her home, her yard, and her gardens. She was a homemaker, finding joy in making fantastic strawberry rhubarb jam, which she bottled in recycled baby-food jars. Our favorite dinners included baked potatoes smothered in margarine, served alongside fresh-cut asparagus from her garden.

She was tall, and as Dad would say, her face was "the map of Ireland." She had big blue eyes, a perfect size-eight figure, and auburn hair that she wore flipped slightly under with the help of her Clairol electric curlers. At 5:00 p.m. every weekday, she would disappear upstairs to wash up from her life as mom and home manager and then reappear back downstairs looking very much like Katharine Hepburn, striking and sweet. With freshly-applied, bright-red lipstick, hair pulled into a soft bun, and a gentle and welcoming smile, the quick-change artist would welcome Dad back from the demands of his day in the newly evolving world of advertising.

When Mom wasn't being a mom she was a community volunteer, taking time to give to those less fortunate than herself. Mom took her charity work with absolute intensity, and we learned not to intrude upon this special side of her.

"Hello. Yes?—wait, let me check." She would open her daily planner during phone calls to see if she was available to help our priest with Mass, deliver meals on wheels, assist homebound seniors, or make a cake for one of our teachers. She never said no, and she never ended a phone call without saying, "Thank you for calling."

Her kindness and energy made her a target, in a way. "Could you…?" "Would it be possible for you to…?" were questions and requests that came at her from many directions. Her answer was always, "Yes, I can."

Every year she was the room mother for each of our classrooms. Seven classrooms equaled seven sets of responsibility and enough brownies baked for what

> **"Her faith was always the answer."**

seemed like half of the school system. She was the volunteer parent who would go into the public elementary and middle schools to lead the children in their walk down the sidewalks to the Assumption Parish Catholic Religion School. I remember being so proud that she was my Mom because she was always so nice to all the kids. If there was one child walking alone, she would ask a random child to take over as leader and quietly fall behind the group and walk with the stray child.

All these things were so typical of Mom; she was always sensitive to the needs of lonely or misunderstood souls and always happy to *give to someone* rather than give to herself. But how did she trust that she would have enough?

Her faith was always the answer. It could not be overlooked.

Mom's spirituality was undoubtedly her bedrock foundation, and she showed devotion by doing.

She was famous in the community for giving fresh, warm, delicious treats to someone who was struggling or suffering. Sliding pans of freshly baked brownies, breads, cookies, or cakes would come out of the oven, and she'd call us into the kitchen, so we could wrap them in plastic and attach a simple note that said, "With love from the McDonough Family." We would all be assigned to get on our bikes and deliver these "love-gifts" to people from church who were ill or others whom she wanted to thank for their kindness to her brood or husband. During Christmas season, we would walk throughout the neighborhood delivering her baked goods to our twenty-five-plus neighbors on her Christmas list.

In the summer months, the smell of her signature cinnamon-apple bundt cake, brought neighborhood kids in from around the block.

"Mrs. McDonough…do you have any cake?" Tenney, my brother's best friend, who basically grew up in our home, would charge through the back door, not saying hello, but seeking one of her warm baked goods.

"On the counter," Mom would tell him, and he would open the drawer, take out a knife, and cut a slab of still-warm cake. The remarkable thing was, Mom would do this with all of our friends. Little wonder our neighbors thought she was special—her spirit shone through everything she did.

Faith in action—that's who Mom was.

For thirty-four years Mom managed her husband and seven children. After Tricia left for college, and with no more children in their home, their lives became even more entwined as one. They continued their nightly rituals of ice cream. They laughed. They traveled through Ireland, and ultimately Mom worked for Dad as his assistant and secretary in his newly found career of professor.

She would take dictation of his teaching notes for his students. The university where they worked, Empire State College, was a mentorship-style university that offered coursework for older students in need of a college degree to advance in their careers. His office, one hallway down from her secretarial desk, was unlike the predictably decorated offices with gray, stainless steel file cabinets and matching gray, stainless steel desks. Dad's office was *different and better*. Dad's office was more of a storyboard collection of their passions.

Different and Better. That's what he taught as his subject matter at college and his home. The office of my father, the professor, had charm and warmth. Like a hideaway, it was in the far corner of the university center and had its own back entranceway from the parking lot. He would welcome his students, often the same age as Dad, and quickly capture them with his wit and fascination for all things from the past. Students would fall into his world beyond academia, as he would engage them with stories, describing in great detail when and where he had found items to add to the collections that adorned his office. He had a gumball machine from the 1940s, and nautical artwork hung all over the walls, celebrating his love for ships and Commodore Nelson. His bookcases housed hundreds of books on creativity, imagination, and the power of the brain. On his bookshelves, he displayed ships in a bottle, many of them his constructions, cast-iron penny banks dating back to 1840, and a glass sculpture of the phrenology of the brain.

From the ceiling hung a three-foot lightbulb that he had jerry-rigged into a ceiling fixture. When his students had a "bright idea," he would turn on the light and celebrate their success. Outside of his office, he had an Irish flag, hanging on a flagpole. As students entered his office, they could find a huge 1940s, seven-foot-tall, white porcelain drug-store penny scale, like the kind seen in a Jimmy Stewart movie. A 1960 solid oak phone booth, (think Clark Kent changing into Superman clothes), was on the left, and hundreds of matchbox cars that he had collected for years, were showcased on his bookshelves. We would visit him in his office, and because we all loved the scale and the telephone booth, once retired, he brought them home to adorn our family kitchen. Yes, we had a 1940 white porcelain penny scale and a telephone booth in our house when I was growing up.

Dad spoke at advertising club luncheons and university professional development seminars extolling the power of creativity and challenging his audience to *think outside of the box*. His students both loved and admired him, and it was with great pride and joy that he would introduce them to our family. His students became his dear friends.

Dad's collections weren't confined to his office. They filled our home well beyond the transitioned porcelain drug-store scale and the 1960s telephone booth. He and Mom spent great amounts of time at art museums, attending art lecture after art lecture, and always left with a piece for her or for them from a particular exhibit. Sometimes it was a poster of an exhibit or a replica piece from the exhibit. It didn't matter to either of them how exciting a piece was to someone else: they collected pieces that appealed to their memories. For Dad, though, this pastime had even more significance.

When he discovered certain treasures, Dad would research their historical significance and use them to open discussions in his creativity seminars. His message was the same to each student, as well as to us: *While things have a value to life, the value of things themselves does not matter. Something that is valuable is so because of its story **and** connection to you.*

That was Dad. Dad's message was the story behind his collections, not the collection itself. That was what his students loved about him. Dad could pick up an object and minutes into his storytelling, the object became a piece of fascinating artwork.

Apart from his far-ranging travels, his teaching, and his community work, there was always only one place Dad would rather be. Dad was happiest when he was just *with her*—his Bernadette—sitting in the backyard or alone with her at the kitchen table. He was grounded in her, relying on her self-taught secretarial skills and her ability to multitask. I remember coming home many Sundays and watching them outside in the backyard near her rose beds. They would sit under a shade umbrella, and he would dictate to her a college memo regarding his sabbatical interest, or she'd check his grammar and spelling on a letter to the newspaper editor updating the village residents on a new and exciting urban renewal project, all while sipping tea and savoring her special cinnamon cake. Notably, when he was with her, there was always calm. He knew he had a treasure in her, and what a treasure she was.

Besides the management skills of a Fortune 500 CEO, she had beauty, efficient typing skills, and the ability to create great recipes and stretch a dollar. Mom was all of this, wrapped around a heart the size of Texas. She was the executive director of his home and had complete responsibility for the academics, social behaviors, and scheduling of his seven children—not an easy part-time job. She loved him, and he loved her. Indeed, there was never a doubt in my mind that his greatest pride was the auburn-haired beauty at his side.

They explored their beloved Ireland and immersed themselves in Irish literature and music. In dedication to their heritage, each St. Patrick's Day he would provide the village DPW with Irish green paint and paint one solid green line all the way from outside of our home to the center of the village.

He continued to express his love for her through his tinkering. When the village was excavating to improve the roadway in front of their home, he convinced the workers to place a boulder found during the excavation directly in front of their beloved house, on the left side of their front entrance steps. A boulder? For what? A love story, we would learn. As a self-taught soldering craftsman, he soldered two

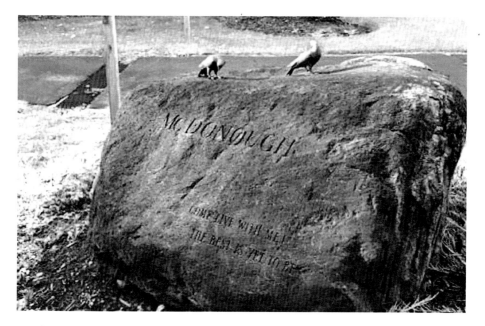

The boulder now sits at the entrance to the cemetery of their parish of 43 years.

love birds on top of the boulder and inscribed into the rock, with his own steady hand, a message of love to his bride: *Come live with me, the best is yet to be.*

They celebrated their fortieth wedding anniversary by renewing their vows at the parish in the village, followed by an intimate reception lovingly hosted at the home of my sister. Our aunts and uncles and all seven of us, along with our children, spouses, and their friends, celebrated their marriage of forty years. A pin drop could have been heard as she entered the renewal of vows mass, forty years later wearing her original wedding dress, unaltered, looking as beautiful as she did when it adorned her lovely figure four decades earlier.

What a treasure he had.

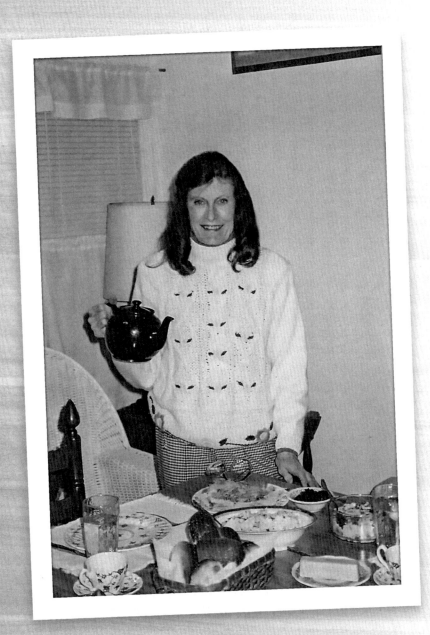

....

CHAPTER 3

That Day

When we were little kids, it was always Mom who was the parent who was most involved in our everyday needs, and when the seven of us turned into parents ourselves, the pattern continued with Mom being the one who would call us and check in on her thirteen grandchildren scattered across the country.

"How are the boys?" No matter how I answered this question when Mom called, and she called at least three or four times a week, she would be elated over everything I told her. "Wow! You must be so proud of them," she'd say as I listed each and every happening in their early teenage lives. I looked forward to her responses to their accomplishments, because without missing a step, she would always end our conversation with "Well, I'm not surprised…just look at their parents." I'd hang up, feeling her warmth like the wrap of an Aran Isles wool shawl—the kind of warmth that a daughter can only feel from the unconditional love from a mom. I knew, because she told me, that she was proud of both Mike and me as parents. How lucky was I that she loved telling me?

But Dad never called. It wasn't like him to want to talk on the phone. The phone call routine was that Mom would call to chat, and then before hanging up, put Dad on the phone, whereupon he'd offer a brief conversation about his latest tinkering projects.

But Dad's calls started coming in pretty regularly after the "no-show beauty parlor day," and his calls were not about his tinkering but his concerns "about your mother."

He was worried that she wasn't interested in the usual things anymore. She wasn't herself. She slept more and wanted to go out less. He worried about all kinds of things, and as much as I am embarrassed to admit it, I thought he was being a bit selfish and particularly harsh on her. After all, she had raised seven kids and put up with all kinds of struggles and demands in her life. *Give her a break,* I thought, completely dismissing his comments. When I'd hang up from his calls, I'd look for something to grab or clench in frustration about his selfishness and angrily tell my husband Mike that "Dad, as usual, was calling about *himself,* not about *her.*" I was sure of it, because when I talked to her she seemed fine.

But then, *that day*, I saw things differently, and I wasn't so sure.

That day. I'd gone to my parents' home at Dad's urgent request to go with him to see a specialist for Mom. I found them sitting at the kitchen table, the same kitchen table where seven nights a week for over fifteen years I sat with my parents, brothers, and sisters and ate dinners of fish sticks, sloppy joes, baked potatoes with margarine, and Friday night clam chowder. Years ago, after the table was clear of dinner dishes, it transformed into an oversized homework desk scattered with books ranging from kindergarten math to English *Regents* prep books. So that she could keep abreast of her household demands, a stack of Dad's laundered shirts and my brothers' Cub Scout uniforms would be piled on a chair at the far end of the table, ready for Mom to iron while she kept a watchful eye on our studying.

At one time, the table had nine slat-back chairs with four extra (for additional drop-in eaters) that were stored in the laundry room next to the kitchen. That day, there were just three chairs: one placed at the head of the table where Dad sat, with one chair on the right-end corner and one chair on the left-end corner, creating the form of a small arch. I was taken aback by the noticeable change as I looked at it that day, remembering that when I was a kid, the table felt huge. My mind flashed back to when all seven of us—nine including Mom and Dad—were piled around the twelve-foot rectangular table. The setting was more like the mess hall from *M*A*S*H* than the all-American family dinner scenes on *The Brady Bunch*.

That day, as I walked in, Dad was hovering over Mom, who was seated in her chair on the left side of the arch. He was coaching her on where the pieces of a makeshift puzzle fit. He had taken an envelope from the mail and cut it into large pieces, handed her Scotch tape, and was gently mixing the envelope pieces on the table in front of her. He was coaching her as she attempted to re-piece the four envelope cutouts into their original form to recreate the envelope.

"Good one! That-a-girl," he was saying, as I walked in the door. It reminded me of the way I spoke to my boys when they were little and learning how to read. Radiating with pride from his acknowledgment, she continued her puzzle, not noticing me as I walked through the door.

Oh, my God. I was seeing first-hand what Dad had been telling me over the last month before the "no-show beauty parlor day." I had ignored Dad's complaints that Mom was not herself, that something about her was not right and that she wasn't as alert as she used to be.

She's just slowing down, for Pete's sake, I had thought.

But now, seeing her lost look behind her little-girl smile as she playfully placed the puzzle pieces, I finally got it. I felt my face tighten up and a huge knot form in my stomach. *What is going on here?*

As I gazed over at them both, I could taste the fear in the back of my mouth. Dad was sitting with Mom, not complaining or pouting about her "lack of…" but broken and trembling. As he reached over to help her with the puzzle, his hand was shaking. This was not the man I knew. I knew him and saw him as strong and tall, long legged, and firm with a handshake that meant, "Let's do business." He was the mayor of our village and was known for refusing defeat. But what I saw that day was a man stumbling, trembling in his words, recognizing his own limitations and fighting hard to not surrender to what he knew he would soon have to accept. He was losing her.

A switch went off in my mind, and I was projected into a setting other than my childhood kitchen. I wasn't watching my mom and dad; I was looking at an elderly man tenderly helping an elderly woman. I was watching their romance story play out in incomparable pain.

Oh, my God. She can't remember how the pieces fit.

It felt like hours before Mom looked over and smiled at me, noticing my entrance for the first time. I wondered as I hugged her with a smothering embrace, "*Is she in pain, or is it just Dad that is in pain? Are they both? Am I in pain or just total confusion? How will I tell this story to my six siblings? Are we all about to see the stealthy progression of what Dad has been telling us and what we (at least I) have only accepted as signs of Mom's simple aging?*"

Dad knew before anyone. Onset dementia was stealing the mind of the one he loved. An enemy that plays by no rules had broken into his world. He had all the play books on how to love her and protect her in any other way, yet there was no play book on how to safeguard her now. He had a plan for their life together, and he was losing. She was his connection to all that was good, and the connection was coming apart.

We put aside the pieces to the puzzle, and I helped both of them into my car. Within the hour we were in the specialist's office, anxious for the appointment that my sister Tricia had secured. Trish, a pediatric neuropsychologist, had reached out to her medical contacts and was able to get Mom on a geriatric neuropsychologist's new patient cancellation list.

SPEAK ~~TO ME~~ OF LOVE

YOUR EYES
TELL ME
AS MINE DO YOU
COMMUNICATE
AS WORDS CAN NEVER DO
OF YESTERDAY
AND LOVE

I could see Dad's anxiety as he fidgeted with her fingers wrapped tightly in his hand while we walked past the office receptionist toward the examination room. "This will be good, Bernadette. He should be able to help us," he whispered to her as he guided her into patient room number one. *Please, God,* I remember praying, still overwhelmed at what I had seen with the puzzle play, *there must be a medicine to help her.*

She accepted Dad's gentle kindness as he helped position her onto the patient chaise. She sat on the edge, her feet adorned in frilly lace ankle socks and white sneakers. She was swinging her feet back and forth like a happy child on an elementary school playground swing set when the geriatric neurologist entered the room and told her she had pretty blue eyes. She smiled shyly and sweetly and let out an adorable child-like giggle that could melt the heart of a tin man.

He asked, "Can you tell me your full name?"

"Bernadette."

"And your last name?"

No answer. A long pause.

"McDonough," she finally said.

"How do you feel, Bernadette?"

A long pause. "I'm good," she giggled, her feet still swinging.

The doctor turned to my father. "Peter, tell me what concerns you about Bernadette's health."

Dad dropped his head and looked at the tile of the office floor, his characteristically tall posture now sagged and hunched over. When we first walked into the physician's room, Dad held his chest high, as if he were a warrior ready to protect his princess. But while the doctor was probing and searching for answers, I noticed a shift in Dad's composure: he was sitting slumped in the chair and holding his head in his hands.

In response to the doctor, Dad listed all the things he had said to me on the phone over the last year or so. "She doesn't do—She's not who she was. She's messy, dirty, unkempt, and not keeping house. She has no interest in eating and sleeps late until I have to wake her up."

I was shocked. *How dare he? How could he talk about her like that to a stranger? Mom was sitting right there! Didn't he care that he would hurt her feelings?* My hands turned to fists as I placed them under my thighs. I scrunched my face in anger as I glared at him thinking. *Are you kidding me? How can you be so mean and selfish and talk only about how her aging is affecting YOU?*

I raged inside. This appointment was not supposed to be about him and his need to be taken care of, or about how she was no longer making herself pretty *for him* or doing this or that *for him.* That was how I heard his words, when, in my mind, *we were here to talk about how to help her stay happy and healthy as she aged.*

I continued to glare at him.

"Okay, Bernadette," the doctor said, "I am going to ask you a couple of questions. Take your time answering. Where were you born?"

"New York," she answered.

"Where do you live now?"

"Close to here." Then a moment later, "Fairport."

"What is the name of the president of the United States?"

"Obronga." (She meant Obama.) And she gave a silly laugh when the doctor laughed at the mispronunciation.

"What year is it?" Time lapse. "It's lots of years, I know that," she said, with a sweet tone and happy smile.

Dad remained bent over, looking at the floor.

"What month is it?"

"I don't know, but I know it's winter because we have snow," she replied, again with sweetness in her voice.

"Who is the man next to you?"

"Peter, my husband," she answered, with a giggle like a little girl disclosing the name of her grammar-school crush, rather than the man she was married to for over 55 years.

I would soon learn, all too quickly, that knowing his name and knowing he was her husband was a huge victory in our upcoming journey.

"Who is this girl?" He pointed at me.

"My daughter, Catherine."

I let out a huge breath.

Knowing my name today was another victory for our side.

"Do you have other children?"

"Yes, lots of children."

"How many?" We watched and waited for her to answer. She was wiggling and giggling but offered no response. It was almost as if she was in a wonderland far, far away.

After several long moments of silence, the doctor continued. "Okay, I bet they are all great kids. Let's not worry about how many. Can you tell me their names?"

Time lapse.

I listened anxiously for her response as she searched her mind, gazing up at the ceiling and turning her head back and forth. After a few minutes of silence, she gave three correct names out of her seven children.

The back of my head started to ache, and my hands under my thighs turned clammy with sweat. I shifted in my chair, shocked that Mom couldn't remember all of the names of her seven children.

Oh, my God.

I moved my stare from Dad over to the doctor, who was inputting his notes onto his tablet, seemingly unfazed by her responses—or lack of responses. Dad hadn't flinched.

The doctor continued, "What did you have for breakfast today, Bernadette?"

She giggled. "Well, Peter always makes my placemat with coffee, and a bagel with marmalade." Then she added, "And a napkin."

I would not know the significance of that last, tacked-on item until much later.

Dad knew, though, and I would later wonder if it gave him even the tiniest amount of relief that she had listed it then.

"Does she have Alzheimer's?" I asked the doctor as he moved back to his laptop to input notes.

"No. Alzheimer's is a type of dementia," he answered factually. "Your Mom's dementia, based on her scans and her analysis today, is due to TIA strokes. It's called vascular dementia."

"Strokes?" I gasped. Mom had strokes?

"She might not have known she was having them. TIA strokes are not always felt. They are silent strokes, unlike the strokes one might have in the heart." The explanation ended there.

Oh, my God. Poor Mom.

He gave us prescriptions. One was an antidepressant that also affected memory, and the other pill was specifically useful, when combined with the first, in slowing the progression of memory loss.

Slowing the progression? Does that mean it doesn't cure this? Mom had strokes and we didn't know it? I felt a panic rising in my throat and wanted to scream the questions pounding in my head. *What about stopping the progression? What about bringing her back?*

We needed another doctor. We needed to do something. We needed to take vigorous action.

When we left the office, my hands were still shaking. I was frustrated with Dad, with Mom, with myself, and with this supposedly expert doctor. My mother's mind was vanishing before our eyes. What were we supposed to do now?

Mom was seated in the back seat, smiling out the window like a happy child.

We did the only thing I could think to do, knowing she loved chocolates and desserts. We went for ice cream.

Four months later, we were back with the same doctor in the same office.

He again told her she had pretty blue eyes. She again smiled and giggled, sitting just like she had during the last appointment, although this time getting up onto the chair, she was a bit more unsteady and required the help of us both. Once situated, her feet started to swing, just like in the last appointment, as if she was a toddler back on a swing set.

"What is your name?"

"Bernadette."

"What is your last name?"

No reply.

"Who is the man with you?"

"Oh, that's Peter."

"Who is he?"

Blank stare.

"Who is this girl?" He pointed to me.

Time lapse.

"Catherine."

"And she is?"

Another blank stare. My throat tightened.

The geriatric neuropsychologist would not meet my gaze and continued his assessment when she did not answer his question.

"On this piece of paper, can you draw me the hands of a clock at the three o'clock hour?"

With the pencil cupped by her thumb and three fingers, she awkwardly but happily drew what she knew of a clock. She drew no hands on the clock. She drew the numbers 1, 2, and 3 in the center of the circle. She then skipped all other numbers and drew the number 9, and placed it outside the circle.

I couldn't even look at my Dad. I could barely breathe. Where was Mom? *Where was my mom?*

I dropped my head to my knees and stared at the floor. Dad did the same.

If the day of the "no-show beauty parlor" had been hard, and if *that day* in the kitchen watching her attempt to complete a toddler's puzzle had been terrible, then this day was the worst of them all.

The doctor wrote a prescription for another drug that might offset some of her fatigue and advised us to be patient with her memory loss and monitor her behavior. In other words, he offered nothing new.

When we left his office that afternoon, I knew in my heart that this would be the last visit with that doctor. There was something seriously wrong, and I had to let my siblings know.

Just as we had needed our parents when we were children, now they needed us.

I brought them home, and said I'd stay for a couple of days just to be around if they needed me. Dad refused my offer.

"We'll be OK now that she has new medicine. Thanks for helping. I can take care of things now. You go back home," he said. So I did. I couldn't challenge him and his capability to care for her. I just didn't have the heart or the energy left to say what I knew was the answer to their crisis: *We need to move her into an assisted living center.*

Mom was experiencing mental and physical disintegration, meaning she was losing her connections and her beautiful mind. Dementia was stealing from her a mind that had skipped third grade, graduated from university with honors, and over sixty years before, captured and held my dad's heart.

I returned home that evening and sat with the boys and Mike at our kitchen counter cluttered with an SAT study guide, a history textbook, and a double-cheese pizza that Manny had picked up on his way home from football practice. I quietly watched as the boys studied and ate, all the while wondering: *Would anything in our lives ever be the same?*

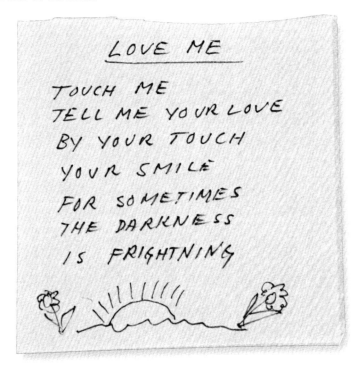

Morning sonnet on a napkin.

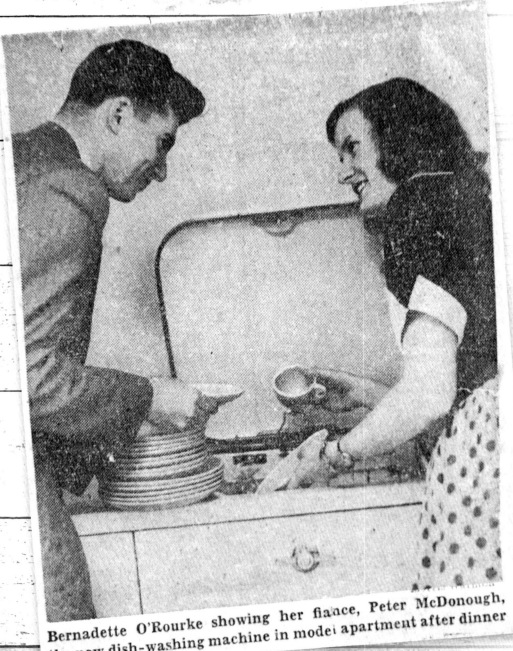

Bernadette O'Rourke showing her fiance, Peter McDonough, the new dish-washing machine in model apartment after dinner

CHAPTER 4

....

His Plan vs. Our Plan

For three long years after the no-show beauty parlor day, her mind continued to disintegrate while the minds of all seven of us became increasingly concerned about how to help them. What was the answer? There had to be a plan. What we found was that there were plans. In fact, all too quickly, we learned of three separate plans: Dad's, ours (the children), and God's.

Plan Number One: Dad's plan. He would build them a fortress.

Although he was not an architect, fear of the future and dementia's swift progress, ignited my dad's genius. He designed for them a retirement condominium, with special accommodations for Mom, located just one quarter-mile from my own home. As with everything in their lives together, this was typical of my father. He had an answer, and control of all things, for both of them. Or so he believed.

His challenge at that time was how to stay together and out of nursing care. What he wanted was to build a fortress that would protect her against the disease closing in on them.

And so he focused his energies.

He loved working on his blueprints: one floor, walk-in bathtub, seated shower, motion lights along the baseboards of every room, and no steps for her to trip on when entering from the garage. He found the best prices for appliances that had emergency shut-off valves in case she forgot she had turned something on—the oven, stove top, coffee maker, toaster, or her Clairol electric curlers. The blueprint included no doors, just extra wide entrances separating the rooms in case her future included a wheelchair.

My husband Michael and sons Manny and Marshal, then seventeen and fifteen, were awestruck by his remarkable brilliance and love for her. Dad wasn't driving much by that time, so I would drive out to Rochester and pick them up to spend the weekend with us. The boys would return home sweaty and smelly from their Saturday mornings of football and wrestling practice, throw down their helmets, kick off their cleats, and take a seat at our island kitchen table. Once seated, Dad would share his progress on the drafts of his blueprints, complete with accuracy in measurements for buttresses, entrance-ways, and nautical wall hangings.

"I'm building this for your grandmother. You can see where I raised the microwave from the lower oven to the top oven, because I use the microwave much more than the oven these days," he proudly told his wide-eyed grandsons, knowing that what he had drawn with his own hands was work more associated with the drawings of a tenured architect.

I was impressed, too, but not only because of his vision and architectural skills. I was used to that. Gee whiz, the man was an absolute genius. I was impressed with him because I realized that he was handling Mom's dementia with his own expressions of love, whether the expressions were apparent to me and my siblings or not. I stopped being angry at him when I let myself accept that it was *their* love and *their* relationship. I began to understand "love languages"—the different ways people express love, and expressions that are counted and felt as love by the one receiving them. I no longer judged, but more often prayed that I could push my energies from being angry at his stubbornness, to appreciating the depth of how he loved her.

These kitchen gatherings offered me a glimpse of what I saw as his *higher level of love*. He was willing to relocate to a new town, give up his community presence and friends, and start a new life with her in a new house, built especially for her. He was recognizing his own limitations and putting all efforts into protecting her from danger, and guarding them both against the threat of her removal. He was beginning to accept that she would eventually have to be in "a place" without him.

Sadly, his plan wasn't happening fast enough, and more importantly, his plan wasn't part of a bigger plan, one that was evolving as his children acted with their own language of love. We needed to intervene sooner than the groundbreaking on his new home. All seven of us had learned well from him, so in the spirit of his legacy, we created a plan with a love for them both which was *different and better*.

In November we held a family meeting and talked about the difficulty and pain of witnessing both of our parents experiencing different types of failing health. We all agreed that *helping* them was even more difficult than *watching* them struggle. Dad was in charge and didn't want help. He only wanted solutions without any-one interfering with his plan. We all agreed that although he had created his own solution to build the condominium and relocate closer to me, we needed to change their situation immediately and not wait for the condo. Dad's health was declining rapidly. The perfect storm was brewing with two very fragile parents living on their own. To make things even worse, Dad was becoming more and more defiant and resistant to any of us getting involved.

He refused to have aides come in beyond his own visiting nurses. Four ulcerations had developed due to his multiple-heart related surgeries, including quadruple bypass, stent implants, pacemaker and defibrillator implant. A wound care specialists came weekly to bandage, cleanse and tend his venous ulcers. The ulcerations caused insufferable pain, and four to six times per day he swallowed narcotics—taking a dosage that today would put the prescribing physician in jail. Yet in my Father's mind, as long as he could think, he could fight the pain; and as long as he could fight the pain, he would fight to keep and protect her.

Plan Number Two: *Our* plan.

None of us had been in these waters before. There was no rule book. We decided on a plan to help them and began to navigate the sea in the most loving way we knew how. We had to do it quickly.

I called Dad three days prior to my arrival at their home. Mom rarely answered the phone anymore as dementia started to affect her speech articulation, and she sometimes couldn't get out the word "hello." As part of our family meeting, we had crafted a compelling story of how Mom needed the joy of being in the company of her grandsons, my boys, who knew of this plan as well. My bargaining tool with Dad was for me to take advantage of the most vulnerable part of his life—protecting his wife. And so the phone call took place.

"Great news, Dad," I said, "How about you and Mom come here for a quick vacation? Just for three or four months during the cold, so that I can help you take care of Mom." I glanced at Marshal's varsity wrestling match schedule on the wall knowing that this new plan of ours would limit how many of his matches I would be able to attend. "There's an opening at a seasonal assisted living around the corner, and the boys and I can see Mom every day, just until the winter ends. Mom will love it. She and I can bake, and I can help her find a physical therapist to help her with her balance." I paused and, hearing only silence, continued. "And while I take care of her, you can rest and take care of yourself and spend more time on your blueprints for your new house."

My hand was shaking as I held on to the phone. Of course, it was our intention to never let them return to their home, to keep them with us until well past the winter months, and I think he knew that. But hearing that I was not worried about him—which, of course, was far from true—that in fact, I was just worried about Mom, he conceded.

I could feel and envision him, holding his head in his hands and hunching over, resigned to defeat, as he choked out the words, "OK, we'll come," he said, "but just for the winter, and I need to bring my treasures and ship models with me."

I had to deliberately choose words that didn't sabotage his fortress plan and punch down his pride. It was far from easy because I was not being honest with him. Breathing slowly I said, "Just start labeling things for me to move that you absolutely can't live without for the next three months." I hung up the phone, shoved my own first-born child's college applications out of the way, and broke into tears.

Three days later, I arrived at the home where Mom and Dad had raised us, their home of 45 years. My sister and Hersh, my best childhood friend (better known among us all as Mom's eighth child), along with the movers, loaded the moving truck with my dad's collections and treasures: my parents' first-ever purchase, their walnut dresser; their original 59-year-old bed; the love seat from their engagement; two of Dad's treasured nautical ships; clothes; and a box of things that Dad had labeled "Bernadette Come Live With Me."

It was a torturous two-hour ride to their new temporary living arrangements, and I prayed that God would let me see through the fountains of tears that were pouring from my eyes as I drove. It was just the three of us—Mom and Dad and me. Mom was in the back of my SUV resting her head on a pillow that was protecting the twelve stitches that had been sewn into the back of her head after a fall five days before. Unbeknownst to me, Dad had called an ambulance after she had tripped on a rug in the living room. Typical of his protective behavior, he demanded that, after the physician finished the stitches, they both return home. He would care for her stitches. Of course. That was his plan.

Dad, in the meantime, was in the front passenger seat with a back support brace around his middle to ease the inconsolable pain from a fall he had taken in the bathroom two weeks earlier while trying to pick up a towel. Again, his pattern of care: a call to 911, the hospital, then a refusal to stay and his insistence to return to their home. The back support ran around the middle of his stomach, a stomach that now measured 56 inches, up from a slim 38 inches from a year ago—the weight gain due to massive water retention and over all bad health.

They moved into assisted living two hours later, a half mile from my home, on the same Friday I had picked them up. My best friend Kimmie, Marshal, Manny, and Mike were there to meet us and help get them settled into their new temporary home. Kimmie had organized the apartment with new low mattresses, filled the refrigerator, put Mom's favorite soups in the cabinets, and made sure that Mom's marmalade and bagels were set and ready for her Saturday morning wake-up.

But then the third, unexpected plan surfaced, and it was brutal. An insurmountable challenge reared its head, triggering a cascade of events that threw us all out of control.

Plan Number Three: God's plan.

That Friday evening would be the one, and only night my dad stayed in their new apartment.

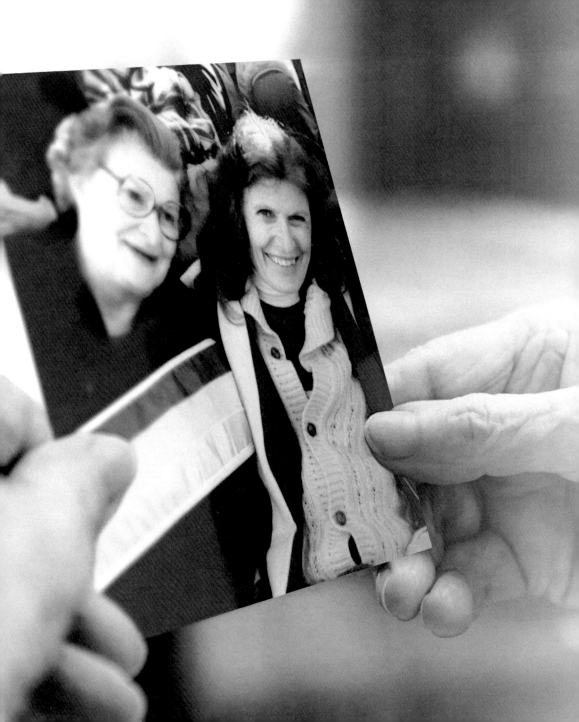

....

CHAPTER 5

Accepting the Unwanted and Unacceptable Things

There is a universality about accepting the role of being a parent to parents, about accepting that our parents will lose the ability to help themselves, about accepting that our parents are no longer who they were, about accepting that there is a resistance when parents do not like their children interfering in their lives. These are all issues faced by those with aging parents. Complicating this further, is when a child is watching a parent disappear into a fog. Having a parent *with* you, but not really *there* with you—that is deep grief.

But add in the need to accept that you are watching someone disappear into an abyss, and one finds that it gets even harder.

I was entering yet another chapter as caregiver into their lives. Neither our priest nor their doctors could give me or my siblings the answers that we needed to prepare us for what was about to happen. We were operating without any handbook.

After all the years of protecting her, and dismissing his own chronic and debilitating pain, Dad stayed only one night with her in their new assisted living home.

We were learning a life lesson aligned with one of my cousin Sidney's most quoted Yiddish adages, *"Mann Tracht, Un Gott Lacht."* English translation: "Man plans and God laughs."

On Saturday morning at 7 am, the day after we moved my parents out of their home of 45 years, I brought Dad to the hospital. He was complaining of weakness and shortness of breath.

He was immediately diagnosed with congestive heart failure and admitted. The E.R. doctors reviewed and questioned his narcotic use, took x-rays, and found that, in fact, he had a broken tail bone and two broken discs in his back. I listened as he weakly told the doctors he'd fallen a month before, how he'd gone by ambulance to the hospital, but had refused to overnight in the hospital and signed himself out in fear of Mom's being left alone at home. Because of this, he was never treated for the injury, left the hospital, accepted new debilitating pain, and returned home to care for her.

I stayed with him in the hospital that Saturday and Sunday night until Monday morning when a neurosurgeon operated on his spine. For three years, he had been on multiple medications, including the heart medicine amiodarone. After his spinal surgery, he experienced a stroke from an amiodarone overdose and was admitted to the ICU. After two weeks in the ICU, he was released into a stroke rehab center. And after three weeks of rehab and very little progress, the facility changed his status and admitted him into their long-term nursing care. After three weeks in the long-term nursing care, I couldn't take anymore and moved him into my own home with the help of hospice.

My parents brought me into this world. It was now my job to help Dad out of his.

It was my turn to reach for a power of love I had never known.

NEW DAY

MORNING
DAY IS   DAWNING
     I CAN SAY
     I LOVE YOU
IF I CAN STOP
   FROM YAWNING
BUT WHAT I SAY
   IS NOT IN JEST
BECAUSE I LOVE YOU
AND WILL
MY WHOLE LIFE THRU

<u>SHORT</u> <u>POEM</u> <u>WRITTEN</u> <u>IN</u> <u>HASTE</u>

TIME IS SHORT
GOT TO RUN
I LOVE YOU MORE
WITH EACH RISING SUN

CHAPTER 6

A Force Greater Than His Love

We were in a race and didn't know it.

Mike, Manny, Marsh, Kimmie, and I helped the medical transport attendant push Dad's gurney through the main front door of our home into the living room on right side of our colonial house. It had been a *living room* to us for eighteen years, and now it was about to become a room in which he could die. *Did that make it a dying room?*

God, help me.

When we said goodbye to the staff at the nursing home, Dad's nurses, doctor, and case worker were confident that his death would not be soon, and that he could still enjoy some moments of cognitive clarity.

"You're doing the right thing, Kate," the nurses told me when I said I no longer wanted him in nursing care and would be taking him home with me.

"Know that your time with him is special, and let us know if you need additional help with hospice."

"How long will he live?" I choked on the question, not really wanting to know the answer and regretting that I had asked the question.

The nurse set down her clipboard and looked directly into my eyes. "No one can ever say when a person will pass, but we believe he still has time to spend with you. It will be a while, not right away."

A while—not right away—that's what they believed. That's what I heard.

They were wrong. He didn't have a while. And my time with him was not special. At least not at first.

I was exhausted and frightened out of my mind. This time with him was special? That's what the nurses at the nursing home told me.

What? Are you kidding me?

With all the painkillers for his black legs, his broken back, his scarcely beating heart, and his constant foot ache, Dad could barely see and talk. As soon as he was lifted off the gurney and onto the hospice bed, he began writhing and moaning in pain and yelping the word "help." He was suffering.

This was not special. This was hard.

To me, special was when Man, Marsh, Mike, and I were on a summer cross-country family trip to Major League Baseball stadiums watching the Cleveland Indians vs. the Seattle Mariners, my son's favorite teams. *Special* was watching them hold their gloves open, praying that a foul ball from one of the major-league players would land in their worn-out Spalding gloves.

That was special—sharing moments with all four of us together. This was nothing like that. This was hard. This was awful. This was responsibility like I'd never felt before. Compounding my anxiety over caring for Dad was the concern of what was happening with Mom. The question haunted me: *What would his passing do to her?*

Did she even know he was dying? Did she know *anything*?

She was seated next to his bed and was gently petting his hand. "Is he OK?" She timidly asked me during his first hour in our home. Her voice sounding as if the *"he"* that she was referring to was a helpless newborn fawn, and she was a young child wishing to nurse the fawn to life.

"Is *who* OK, Mom?" I asked, hoping to hear her say, "Peter, my husband, your father." But that wasn't her answer. She didn't offer a response—just a sigh, a soft smile, and a blank stare.

Oh, my God. I flashed back to our time in the neuropsychologist's office. *She didn't know his name or who he was.*

God, help me, I thought once again.

We would sit with him in our living room, now transformed into a hospice medical setting with needles loaded with morphine, a bedpan, a special recliner chair (which he never used), and a portable hospital bed equipped with special reclining settings so that fluid would not collect in his lungs.

"Do not be afraid," I whispered in his ear throughout that long first day and into the dark night. "Dad, don't be afraid."

He would stare at me, as if I was speaking a foreign language. I would stare back, in a trance, wondering what I could do to help him die in peace.

On the second day of caring for Dad my soul began to shift. The trance lifted, and I felt myself enter a new setting—not a hospice setting, but something different.

Something was happening between Dad and me. I could feel from his body that Dad was trying to tell me something. There was something that he needed me to hear. It was different than the messages he sent me from the days of my childhood. It was eerie. I had lived my life with this man as my father, but now I heard him need me to be *more than a daughter to him.* I felt him pleading with me to understand that he needed to meet with my soul and form with me a new type of friendship, the kind that so many long for. A friendship that relies on a secret language shared and understood only between two people.

He was asking me to feel and understand his need to keep protecting her, even upon his passing. I was drawn into a conversation with him by a mystical pulling to *hear* him, without the use of words. He was inviting me to enter his spiritual journey in leaving Earth, and share with me a new language that was just between him and me. It was another language without words—much different, but similar, I realized, to the love language that he shared with Mom when we were little. Through his eyes and the magnetic feel of his soul, *I felt what he wanted me to hear.*

I am afraid, but not of dying. I accept my own death. But when I go, I can no longer protect her—the dwelling in my soul, the only person who has ever truly understood and accepted my shortcomings and faults yet celebrated my wit and mind, the one who never criticized, never doubted, and showed me only gratitude, love, admiration, and respect.

No one understands what she needs. Who will shelter her, know how to love her, care for her, make her toast with marmalade every breakfast? Dementia has stolen so much of her mind that she is now a shadow of herself. Without my voice to speak for her, who will make sure that she does not end up alone, fading away in a nursing home?

As I looked at him, helplessly tucked into the hospice bed, my heart opened up to the voice of his soul. I cared about him and how much he loved her. I cared that they had something that few people ever know. He was dying, and he was going alone, leaving her behind. For him, this was the most unbearable pain.

The doctors and nurses told me that hearing is the last of the senses we lose. So again, I shifted my prayers from wishing for him to be healed to praying that he would understand that I was hearing him. I prayed that he could hear that the messages he was sending me through the language we now shared, a language without words, were coming through loud and clear.

I stopped saying *do not be afraid* and stepped away from hovering over him. It was their private time together, and I began to watch and listen to the two of them from a distant chair that Mike had put in the adjoining sunroom. The day room was bright, but the silence from his hospice room was as quiet as the darkness of night. The only sound was the synchronized cadence of their breathing. Each hour, I excused myself for interrupting their peaceful rhythm and shifted his body so that he wouldn't develop painful bed ulcers. I didn't let on to him that I was exhausted and scared. I was simply sad as I watched their love story unfold in front of my eyes—the old fashioned kind of love story shaped by sharing a world for six decades.

That night when the night nurse arrived, I didn't say goodnight to Dad and tell him how much I would miss him. That's what I used to say to him when I would say goodnight to him at the nursing home. But now our soul language told me he didn't want to hear those words. He needed to hear something that had much more meaning to him than my missing him.

Holding his hand and laying my head near his ear, with tears pouring down my face, I whispered to him, "Thank you, Dad, for all the love you have given to Mom your whole life. It must have been so painful to watch dementia close in on her. I am so sorry, Dad, that I wasn't listening. I didn't *hear* you tell me how sad and scared you were. I wish I had listened, Dad. I wish I had listened much sooner than I did."

In our own newly formed language, I felt him message me back. "It's OK." I heard his words through the tender movement of his fingers that were wrapped in mine.

A shiver shot up my spine. He'd heard me. Our language was working.

For five days, he simply rested. No food. Cloth baths. Mom stayed at his side and continued petting his hand, reminding me of a child petting a little kitten.

Next to Dad's bed in the makeshift hospice room was the little love seat from their bedroom of 59 years. I had moved it during the original move from our childhood home to their assisted living, when Dad insisted that it be packed with them.

I remember when we were little sitting on it in their bedroom at night, watching TV with him. It wasn't a very comfortable love seat. There were no fluffy cushions, and the armrests were as hard as rocks, but it was something that mattered to them. It was the love seat that was in Mom's parents' home. It was the love seat that she sat upon as Dad got down on one knee and proposed marriage.

To them, it was a piece in time that represented the *beginning* of their life story. I watched her as she was sitting on it now, her small, fragile hips on its edge, leaning over the hospice bed with her head down on the chest of his barely beating heart.

I felt his soul message me a *thank you* for bringing the love seat here for her now. Now, as their life story was turning the corner toward its *ending*.

Hospice taught me how to administer morphine to reduce the severe pain of dying. I never thought I could be strong enough to position the morphine syringe in the back of Dad's left cheek pocket every four hours. As Mom watched me, I wondered if she knew that the man in the bed was dying and that I was helping him in his passage by giving him narcotics to ease the pain of death.

I remember watching her when I opened his lower lip with my left hand, holding the morphine drop in my stronger right hand. The drops weighed less than an ounce, but the weight of what I was doing, helping Dad die, took every ounce of my spirit and physical strength.

Yet amidst my overwhelming dizziness with the reality of what I was doing, there was something tugging at me, telling me that I'd been shown this type of strength a long time ago.

I jolted with the flashback. I was doing *what I had learned by Mom's example—I was doing what had to be done.*

The boys were little, about three and five, when my mom's best friend, her sister Margaret, became very ill.

"It's Mom," she said. I listened to her voice on my answering machine as the boys threw their empty lunch boxes on the kitchen counter. She didn't sound right. "Aunt Margaret called and asked me to come down and stay with her a bit. She's not feeling well. Daddy will be home alone for a couple of days. Can you please check in on him?"

Mom was on the plane to her sister Margaret's the next morning.

When she arrived at Margaret's Jackson Heights apartment, the door to the apartment was unlocked, as if Margaret was expecting her. Mom walked in, and gently yelled out, "Hello, Margaret," waiting to be greeted with her sister's embrace. Instead, she found her older sister on the white-and-black tiled bathroom floor nearly unconscious. Mom called for an ambulance, rode with Margaret to the hospital, and was met by their other sister, Catherine. Four days later, Catherine and Mom stood together as Mom signed the papers to release Margaret from life support. Margaret had succumbed to pancreatic cancer, which she had kept a secret from her sisters.

I remember, at that time, thinking that the reality of what Mom had to do and the responsibility of doing what her sister requested must have been overwhelming, yet, in the hour of need, she'd had the strength *to do what had to be done.*

A staunch Irish Catholic woman, Mom helped Margaret with the faith that she would journey on to perpetual life, a journey in which Mom and Margaret both devotedly believed.

It was my turn now, and "overwhelming" didn't even touch the depth of my fear or anxiety, yet I was doing what Mom herself had done.

I was assisting Dad in his journey—a journey in which he and I both devotedly believed. I quickly learned that there was one particular character strength I needed to find within me: being able to do what has to be done.

Late Friday evening, five days into his hospice care, I heard him mumble, "Miss O'Rourke."—It broke my heart that his mind and soul were flashing back to the days when he would wait for the "pretty Irish lass," Bernadette, at the bottom of the B. Altman's elevator.

He shook and exhaled a loud rattling noise like a snore, and for the first time a force greater and more powerful than his love for his wife entered the room.

"Safe travels, Dad. I will take care of her," I said.

The following day, the Irish flag was flown at half-mast in the village of Fairport.

> TOMORROW
>
> I LAY IN THE DARKNESS
>
> UNABLE TO OPEN THE
> CURTIN TO SLEEP
> THINKING
> OF YOU AND YESTERDAY
> GRIPED BY A FEAR
> THAT YOU MIGHT
> NOT BE NEAR
> WHEN I NEED YOU
> TOMORROW

BERNADETTE
YOU ARE THE WIND
UNDER MY WINGS
THAT LETS ME SOUR
BEYOND
TOMORROW.

YOU KNOW
WITHIN YOUR HEART
YOU WILL ALWAYS
BE MY SWEATHEART
AN NO OTHER

WILL BE MINE
SO I SAY TO THEE
~~COME~~ STAY LIVE WITH ME
THE BEST IS TRULY
~~IS~~ YET TO BE

CHAPTER 7

Different and Better

I t took me quite some time and many sleepless nights after Dad's passing before the complexities of who he was, and the intricacies of their private love language, would come together for me like the pieces of a complex jigsaw puzzle.

Once the seven of us were out of the house, their onetime busy home became naturally quiet. For all the years we were growing up, it was Mom who was up at the crack of dawn making sure all was set for breakfast, lunch, and dinner. But once we were grown and had left home, with no kids to tend to, she slept in a little longer, and it was Dad who was the first one up.

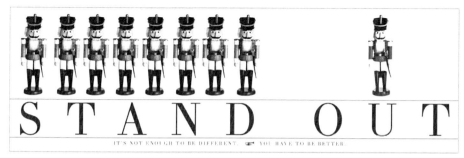

STAND OUT

IT'S NOT ENOUGH TO BE DIFFERENT. YOU HAVE TO BE BETTER.

The banner that hung in the kitchen as a reminder to all seven children.
Stand out. It's not enough to be different. You have to be better.

Every morning, without skipping a day, he'd go downstairs, set her Irish *claddagh* breakfast placemat with a plate, a fork, and a spoon and make a pot of coffee. When she'd come down for breakfast, his magical expression of love would begin.

With nurturing kindness, he'd serve her a cup of coffee with a perfectly toasted poppyseed bagel, spread with just enough margarine to cover the outer circle, and most importantly, pile it with heaps of marmalade to sweeten any dryness. He would saunter over to the kitchen hutch they'd kept since the Cincinnati move and bring her one of his special creations: an orange prescription vial filled with M&M's and relabeled "Daily happy pills for Bernadette." He'd place the vial to the left of the coffee cup so that she could enjoy her dose of chocolate happiness with her last sip of coffee.

To me, this morning ritual sounded like the epitome of kindness and love—a man taking such sweet steps to make his wife happy, by making her a daily breakfast of her favorite things.

But for my Dad, it was not enough. He did more.

We grew up with lots of pictures and hangings throughout our house. Many hangings were replicas of antiques and collectibles, many of them were spiritual, and many were nautical. But one of the most important hangings was a banner that Dad hung in our kitchen, across from the twelve-foot-long kitchen table, above all the seven portraits of his children. The poster was of eight toy soldiers, standing side by side, all the same color, all the same salute. The ninth soldier is separated from the first eight and is standing out in a different color, with a different salute. We all loved that poster with the slogan "Stand out. It's not enough to be different. You have to be better." Growing up in that house, it was the foundation for motivational success: a constant reminder to never stop looking for different and better ways to solve problems and to never quit or give in.

The poster was hung prominently in the kitchen for us all to see and remember, but as Mom's dementia progressed, I think it triggered Dad's creativity and reminded him that his wife needed action that was unique, different, and better than what medical science was offering. He needed to act exactly as he had all of his life—*different and better.*

So, to show his love and devotion for his beautiful wife, Dad provided more than the simple preparation of her morning breakfast. He crafted a morning routine that was *different and better.* Beyond serving her "Daily happy pills," Dad wrote her poetry—daily proclamations of his love, written on a generic napkin, in either red or black marker, seven days a week.

He was a man in love.

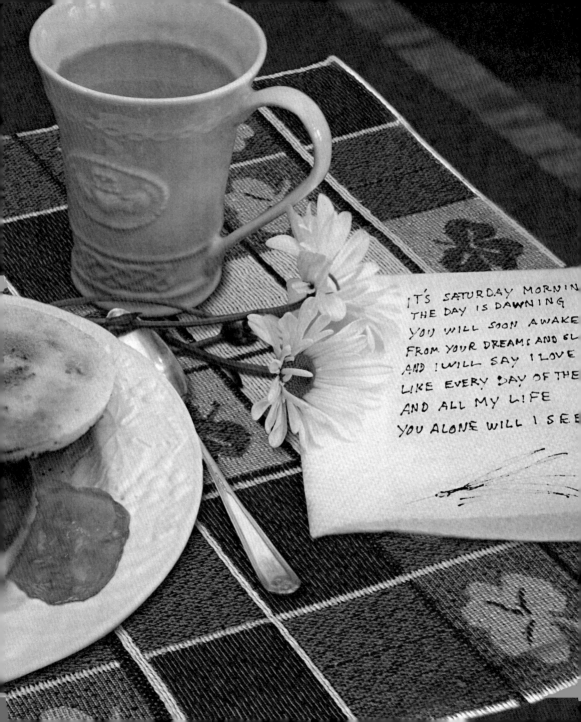

IT'S SATURDAY MORNIN
THE DAY IS DAWNING
YOU WILL SOON AWAKE
FROM YOUR DREAMS AND SL
AND I WILL SAY I LOVE
LIKE EVERY DAY OF THE
AND ALL MY LIFE
YOU ALONE WILL I SEE

CHAPTER 8

....

The Napkins

One of the gifts that I received before Dad died was that he was able to tell me about his fears and his hope that Mom remembered him after he died. During many of my hospital visits to him, he would reflect on the story of his daily napkin writing and breakfast preparation for her. He told me of his napkins and the other poems in the house that were his message to her and to all seven of us, the message that he loved her, always and in all ways, both for who she was and for the magic she brought into his life. He never wanted any of us to forget that, especially Mom. His poems were from the heart, back to the days of ice cream and Central Park and their dreams of the two of them sailing the world. He was a man of true brilliance with no hesitation to write, even with his poor spelling, about the love he felt for his beloved wife.

In our conversations he told me that she would read the napkins, touch them, and then gently kiss him, delighted that she was still the center of his world. So that she would not just read but *feel* his love in the napkins, she would tenderly press the napkin with her right-hand fingers. He would then place each napkin to her right side and his left, so that it sat in front of both of them. The careful positioning assured that the marmalade and her coffee did not spill onto his written promises and sonnets of never ending love.

After breakfast, before the day continued, one of them would pick up the napkin sonnet and place it in a baggie in the drawer of the kitchen hutch.

That's where they stayed until the day I found them.

EACH MORNING
JUST AS DAY IS DAWNING

I BOUNCE OUT OF BED
WITH A POEM IN MY HEAD

AND MAKE THE COFFIE
        AND TOAST

AND A SHORT POEM I HOPE
WILL SAY HOW I LOVE YOU
THAT
        WITH A LOVE THA IS TRUE
        AND ETERNAL TOO

                OVER→

SO FORGIVE MY SPELLING
IT'S ONLY MY LOVE
I AM TRYING AT TELLING

CHAPTER 9

Her without Him

After Dad died, my sweet mom stayed at her assisted living apartment. She never went back to our family home. We sold her house and all the things inside it.

Her downhill slide continued.

Within six months, I moved Mom from the original assisted living apartment into long-term care. Dementia had progressed, and her mind was continuing to weaken, but physically she was still walking and eating. In the aftermath of Dad's death, it was like watching a repeat of her response when Aunt Margaret had died. What was this powerful connection between the sadness in her soul and the progression of dementia?

Watching Mom in long-term care broke my heart. If you are a daughter or son who has a parent with dementia, most likely you know exactly what I mean.

I felt as if no *facility* (a word I hate) was good enough to care for my mom. Although she had the finest and most devoted nurses, doctors, and caregivers, I felt a neverending hopelessness that I was not doing my best, when my best was all I could do. It's awful to feel so helpless.

I had taken on the responsibility of providing care for the woman who gave me life and had promised my dad that in his absence, I could and would provide a happy life for her, and I felt like I was failing. I couldn't stand to find her in the silent setting of long-term care, where she had to smell antiseptics all day and night instead of the peonies and roses she loved. I couldn't stand that Mom was surrounded by patients with levels of acuity much greater than hers. Long-term care was not a fit for her. Mom had life! She had her health. She could walk and sing and smile and give the warmest and most gentle hugs. She just didn't have her memory.

"Your Mom is watching TV."

Almost every time during the three months Mom was in long-term care, when I would go to visit her, the nursing staff would greet me with the words, "Your mom is watching TV." I'd find her in the "great room" in front of the television. But she was not exactly watching TV. In fact, I would find her with her eyes closed, napping, with the TV on channel 66, Turner Classic Movies, mostly from the 1950s and 1960s, all in black and white.

"Hi, Mom! What are you watching?" I'd ask, walking over to where she was slouched over in the chair and waking her up. She never answered the question. I don't think she ever knew and couldn't have cared less. Mom never liked TV. She liked music and activities and caring for people and conversations and singing and baking.

"Well, hello! How are you today?" she would reply, sweetly giggling at the attention she was getting from—who? Who was I?

She didn't know, and frankly I barely even knew my role anymore. I hated that she didn't know I was her daughter, and I hated that I felt so helpless. Each time I would go to pick her up, I would ask her the same question.

"Would you like to go with me and make a cake?"

"Oh, yes, of course. Can we eat the cake?" was always her reply, perking up in her seat and smiling with the same beautiful smile of yesteryear. How could dementia be so mean to a person who was so kind?

Poor Dad, I thought. He'd seen this longer than we had. My heart ached for what he must have felt watching the progression of her disease. My heart and stomach tugged with my own guilt that I'd been so angry at him for being frustrated with her. I wished for something that could not be; I wished I could tell him again how sorry I was for not understanding his pain.

A stab of angst went through me. I was letting my father down.

"Let's go make cake and eat ice cream."

After I signed her out, we'd walk to the car, open up the door, and ever so gently, I'd swing her legs in and buckle her up. I'd turn on the CD of her church music and look up to heaven to pray for—what? Less confusion? Less guilt that I wasn't doing enough because I wasn't doing everything humanly possible to care for her like Dad did? I guess I was looking up for answers.

Dad, I don't know what to do. I'm scared just like you were. There is no peace in my heart. I am afraid because I am out of answers. I don't know what else to do.

Many days, I would take Mom home. I'd strap her into the kitchen counter chair using Dad's old waist harness so that she wouldn't fall, and we would make her famous Duncan Hines brownies. I'd hand her a spoon to stir the brownies, and she would sit and use the spoon to mix the air, never getting the spoon into the batter bowl.

"Way to go, Mom! Marshal will love these," I'd say as she continued to joyously wave the spoon through the air, looking more like the conductor of the Philharmonic Orchestra than a person mixing brownie batter.

It didn't matter that she wasn't really mixing the brownies. I didn't care. I was playing the role of Dad, trying to ignite a memory in her with the smell of the chocolate dessert, hoping that she would be reminded of years past, when she would bake to her heart's content.

"It smells like brownies. Was Grandma here?" Marsh asked one day as he came out the front door and met me in the driveway. I had just brought Mom back to long-term care and packed the brownies with her for the nurses.

With tears streaming down my face, I told him yes, that Grandma had been there, knowing how happy Mom would be to know that he connected her to the smell of warm brownies.

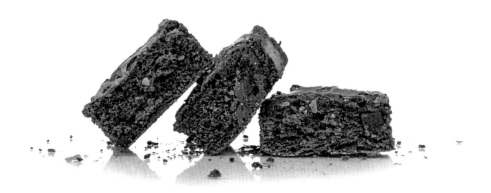

There were times when I knew I had to lighten up a little, so I'd grab on to one of my mom's sayings from our childhood days. When we were little, if she was in a pinch or listening with compassion to a person experiencing hardship, she'd say, "With the help of God, this too shall pass." During my own frustrating moments of despair I would repeat her line and add, "…and *now* would be good."

I could not find peace. I had watched my father struggle against dying because he feared that without him at her side she would spend her life wasting away in a nursing home.

He was right.

I couldn't stand it, and after three months in the long-term care facility, I again moved my mom. This time the move was four miles away from my home to a senior living center that specialized in dementia care. The facility was a one-building structure similar to a home setting, with individual apartments and a circular flow. Residents could walk inside the carpeted loop that went around and around and around and walk in circles until they were exhausted. The facility focused on social interaction, which is what motivated me to move Mom there. I believed in my heart that she would benefit from being with women similar to herself—loving women, who, aside from the cognition and memory loss, were otherwise physically healthy. I wanted her to be with me, but she couldn't have this type of social interaction if she moved in with us.

This move was number four for Mom within two years, and once again, Mike, Manny, Marsh, my friend Richard, and I loaded up a moving van and moved all of her original furniture, including the bed from their original apartment, their Cincinnati hutch, her love seat from their engagement, Dad's huge ships, the portraits of her seven children, piles of photos of her with her grandchildren, and her wedding album to yet another new care center. We brought a continuous-play CD player with her church hymns and her Irish ballads and made sure that the aides in the kitchen served her marmalade each morning. Overall, in her new place we recreated her home that we shared growing up in order to help her retrieve memories of who she had been.

For me, that was the hardest part of dementia. Mom's caregivers never knew the woman inside the body that they cared for. They didn't know the CEO, the community outreach liaison, the church representative, the mom of seven children, nor the person of perpetual peace. They were introduced to the new woman whose behavior and mannerisms were as adorable as a little four-year-old girl's. They were naturally smitten by her, but it broke my heart that I couldn't help her be respected as the remarkable woman I knew her to be.

My brothers and sisters visited Mom and took her on day trips. I suppose we all felt it was easier on us to not sit with her in her "dementia home," but instead to be with her somewhere else, just one on one, hoping in private for a glimpse of the past her.

I'd take Mom anywhere I could—anything to get her out of the dementia home, anything to keep her as my mom, and anything to keep my promise to my dad to protect her. She was darling as we walked the grocery aisles, me with my arms wrapped around her letting her push the cart, allowing the cart to act as her walker. On Sundays, I'd pick her up for church, and so she wouldn't have to walk up to the altar, the priest would come to her in the front pew and present her with the Host. When my sister, Mary Margaret, would come to see Mom, they'd sing rounds and rounds of *Oklahoma* the lyrics of which, for some reason unbeknownst to us, our mom remembered. After *Oklahoma* the two of them would break into her church songs together, repeating the same verse of "Make Me A Channel of Your Peace," again and again until well into the evening. Everyone was so sweet to her, seemingly knowing that kindness was the best medicine for her memory.

Every one of my girlfriends, many of whom had already lost their own mothers, opened their hearts and souls to help by visiting and always including her in invitations for dinners and holidays. I'll never forget the day I relayed a conversation I'd had with Mom after yet another frustrating and exhausting day to my compassionate friend, Ann.

Mom and I had taken a road trip to Poughkeepsie, New York, about four hours from our home. We were driving back from seeing her brother-in-law, Thomas, her sister Catherine's husband, and a terrific group of my cousins, all of whom knew Mom to be one of the world's greatest aunts. As usual, Mom was happy and sweet, although she didn't remember who any of the relatives were. Yet something in the visit with them must have triggered a memory from her past, because on the drive back, she awakened from her cat-nap and blindsided me with a question.

"Do I know your mother?"

I couldn't breathe. My eyes welled to the point of tears, blinding my vision. There was so much pain in that question, and to the answer to that question. What was happening? I knew she didn't know me, but it had never hit so hard before. *I shouldn't be driving,* I thought. *I need air. I need my husband. I need my sons. I need my sister. I need someone to understand—I need my father.*

I took a moment to answer, as she stared at me with her beautiful, innocent smile.

"Yes," I said, finally. "You do know my mother, and she is beautiful, and I love her." I looked out the window, took in a big breath, and turned my head back to her. "You are my mom," I said to her.

She didn't reply.

Rolling down the window did not offer me enough air to pull me out of the reeling pain of her question. Thank God for New York State Thruway stops. I pulled over at the first one and bought a large ice cream with two spoons. Mom and I sat without talking, as I spooned the ice cream past her tender, thin lips; all the while, tears poured down my face.

Weeks later we sat on her love seat in the dementia facility, and I told her what her life was like: that she was a beautiful woman named Bernadette. She had seven incredible children who adored her and a handsome husband named Peter. She sat quietly for a bit, her legs crossed and knees swinging side to side. She giggled.

"You remind me of one of my daughters," she told me, "but I don't know which one."

I thought, *and now would be good.*

But not all of her questions provoked such pain and sadness. In fact, there were moments when Mom's dementia brought me to tears with laughter.

One day we sat together in silence staring at the many photo pages of her seven children and her husband. With each picture, I'd review the names of her children, what they were doing in their lives, and how much each of them loved her. It had to be a full five minutes after the review of each of her children when my sweet mom, true to the soles of her first-generation Irish Catholic toes, asked only one question.

"Did any of my children become a priest or a nun?"

Oh, my God. Finally a moment of grace, levity, and assurance. That simple, single question proved that she, the Irish Catholic mom of my childhood, was still here in my presence, as tender and committed to her faith as ever.

"Hardly, Mom," I answered. And left it at that.

Only God knows where this question came from. Maybe dementia wasn't such an enemy, because clearly she did not remember all the torture the seven of us put her through. For her to think that one of her brood was called and made it through to serve the Church? Wow! Clearly, she had lost her mind.

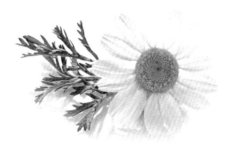

ON A SUNDAY MORNING

YOU ARE REMARKABLE
I AM ALWAYS A STUDENT
LEARNING FROM YOU
THE SPIRIT OF LIFE
TO KNOW YOU AND
LOVE YOU
IS A GIFT FROM ABOVE
SO IN THIS POEM
OF THE MORNING
HERE IS MY LOVE

FAIL

THOUGH TIME
GOES FAST
AND PROBLEMS
COME TOO
MY LOVE
WILL LAST
AND ONLY
FOR YOU

I love you

ROSES ARE
VIOLETS ARE
YOU ARE
CUTEST

....

CHAPTER 10

Dementia Loses Its Fight to the Power of Love

One way that dementia kills our loved ones is by stealing their memory of how to eat and how to swallow, which eventually leads to organs, shutting down.

And that, in fact, was how Mom died.

Dementia stole her from us, yet I now know that in the end of Mom's life, dementia did not win. In fact, dementia lost an important battle during its attack on her.

Mom stayed happy.

I believe it was because of Dad. He spent many years—how many, we will never know—planning how to beat this disease, as he watched it take away his best friend. Dad personalized dementia as the one and only enemy in his life, and made it his fierce goal, to his last breath, to remind Mom what they both believed: *They were one, connected by perpetual memories of love within their souls.*

He never stopped showing her that she was special, that her happiness and comfort meant everything to him, *that her life mattered.* Every day, he repeated his love for her through his written love sonnets. It was their routine, and he orchestrated this daily ritual, praying that its repetition would cement in her mind the love that he had for her, a love never to be forgotten.

Dementia didn't win the entire war. She did keep a memory, but not because of advances in medical science that focus on MRI results and million-dollar technologies and drugs. She kept a memory because of the power of love—my dad's love. He weakened dementia's power by strengthening her soul's memory. He used the power of his own brilliant mind and battled against the disease that was determined to remove him in his starring role in the life they shared.

After my dad died, we cleaned out our family house, packed with things from seven children over forty-five years. We knew Mom would never live there again, and none of us was interested in keeping the house. We were all well established in our own homes throughout the country.

And then came the day…

My sister, my best friend Hersh, and I were cleaning and throwing things out of my parents' home when I opened a cabinet drawer, and I lost my breath, awestruck by the treasure lying before me.

Inside the drawer, just as he had told me during my hospital visits with him, I found a collection of his devotion to her, jewels of love from his heart, evidence of his desire to prove to her that, no matter her memory loss, they were still Peter and Bernadette—two hearts and souls brought together as one. This devotion to her was striking and beautiful yet still so mysterious.

I found letters from 1946, wrapped in an ice cream carton, that my dad had written to Mom while he was in Sampson Naval Base. I found another box titled,

"Come Live with Me." In it was the top of my parents' wedding cake, my baby brother Jamesy's baby shoes, a perfectly organized list of their wedding gifts and attending wedding guests, pictures of their courtship, and pictures of their trips to Ireland.

Most amazingly, there was a gallon freezer bag, with the stacks of napkins he'd told me about. The napkins were neatly folded and placed within the bag, exactly as he described.

Oh, my God. Here they are. I placed my right hand on my heart as I saw the pile of daily poetry written and dated proclaiming his love for her, and of his fight to remind her of their love as they both battled against her disease.

I leaned onto the counter for support with my hands on my head. I remembered the conversations with Dad during his hospital and long-term care, telling me about the sentiments of the napkins and what joy he had in writing for her what he called his "sonnets." Because I was so distracted by my role as caregiver for his pain and medical frailties, I paid those conversations little attention.

A flash of a memory brought me back into the past as I looked at the stack of sealed napkins. I knew these napkins. I had seen his morning setup and kindness to her as she sat down at her spot at the kitchen table on my overnights at their home during the years of their declining health. I remember specifically one morning, when I saw a sonnet at the table and told Dad that I thought it was so sweet. He gently smiled

The top of their wedding cake found next to the ice cream carton and morning napkins

73

and did not reply—as if it were private between them, not for anyone else. These were the secrets of his heart. He didn't boast of the sentiment written on the napkin sonnets. He didn't comment on the writing from his soul. He didn't comment on their life together. He didn't bring me into the intimate conversation of what was written from him to his love. Their love language belonged only to them.

Seeing the collection that day magnified the new lens I used in viewing their marriage and our lives as a family. I remember feeling an even stronger commitment to keeping my promise to Dad by making Mom as happy as I could, especially without him there.

No wonder she was so darn happy. For me, I had just found the secret to my mom's continued state of peace and everflowing sweetness: She had been loved.

I took the pile of sonnets, the trinkets and photos in the box labeled "Come Live with Me," and headed back home to my mom, my sons, and my husband.

—•◦•◦•—

During her time at the dementia care home, Mom was served her daily breakfast in the main dining room of the home. A caregiver would awaken her in the morning, cleanse her, and brush her auburn hair before walking her to her designated breakfast spot. Things were going as well as things could go until Mom stopped eating.

The call came around 9:30 on a Monday morning, just after her morning breakfast ritual.

"Kate, we're concerned about your Mom. Lately, she just seems lost at breakfast." I put down my coffee and leaned against the kitchen wall. "Other meals seem OK, but we are considering changing her schedule and needed to let you know."

She went on to explain that sometimes with dementia patients, sleep schedules and internal clocks switch, and that may be what Mom was experiencing. "It may be best to let her sleep through breakfast," she suggested. "She just sits and stares at her placemat, and looks into the air and seems to pet the table napkin."

All I heard was the last sentence. Chills ran down my spine, and it was as if my father was standing in the room next to me.

Dad. I said to myself. *Dad, she needs you.*

She's looking for Dad's napkins…She remembers something…Oh, my God…She remembers something!

I knew what I had to do. With the stack of the sonnet napkins in Dad's moving box labeled "Come Live with Me," I drove through the back roads to the dementia facility.

I walked in holding Dad's box as if the box held a newborn baby. I found Lynda at the nurse's station and took the bag of napkins out of the box. I carefully placed the bag down on the counter and explained that this bag of napkins was more than just that. What I'd brought was the outpourings of my dad's heart. I explained how he'd written these poems each and every morning and how they sat next to Mom's breakfast plate. Reluctantly, I pulled the top napkin from the bag. And I watched as Lynda's eyes read the poem and filled with tears.

She took my hands into hers. "Kate," she said, "Can I put these in a remembrance book for your mom? Then we can place it next to her every morning at breakfast." I nodded and let the tears fall down my face.

That night when I returned home to Mike and my sons, there was a message on the answering machine from the nurse at the dementia home.

Kate, I just wanted to tell you that your mom seems great. I was with her tonight and put her remembrance book next to her place setting. As we turned through the pages of the book, your mom was giggling, putting her hands on the pages and petting the napkins with her fingers. It was so wonderful! I put the machine on pause and screamed for Mike and the boys to come and listen. We stood side by side letting it play from the beginning and heard the rest of the message: *It feels like she's actually interested in reading and touching the napkins. It's almost like she's searching for someone—your dad, maybe? Anyway, Kate, she's happy again. She ate all of her chicken soup and had ice cream for dessert.*

And so it became part of Mom's daily ritual to sit and "read" the napkins. She no longer just sat at breakfast—she ate and smiled. She still didn't know who she was or where she was, or that I was her daughter. She no longer knew she had other children, who longed for her to be their mom again. But she did remember something. Through the napkins she remembered happiness and she remembered her husband.

He didn't lose her.

Dementia had won the blue-ribbon prize physically—but my dad's love, in poetic words, had beaten dementia at its own, unfair game. Mom *remembered* that somewhere, at some point, these napkins comforted and warmed her mind, body, and soul.

Checkmate, dementia. You lose.

....

CHAPTER 11

And the Greatest of These Is Love

A s the end came near—

The napkins restored Mom's memory. I still cry as I realize the power of Dad's poetry. He did it. Dad won the battle in his personal war against dementia. She did not forget him.

But the disease continued its blows. All seven of her children watched dementia's progressive path, and we mourned the loss of the special, unconditional feeling of love that Mom gave to each one of us throughout our lives. It was simply sad. We missed her even though she was still with us.

Yet inside this remarkable woman, we were to learn of an internal battle that must have been brewing between Mom's soul and her mind. We heard something incredible as Mom fought to come out of the abyss of dementia and say goodbye to each and every one of us. She was going to do *what had to be done*: she was going to assure her children that her starring role of motherhood, in each one of our lives, was far from forgotten.

— Two months later —

Hospice told us that her time was quickly approaching, and my brothers and sisters responded immediately to my phone calls telling them that it was likely that Mom would pass within days. Each of them came within hours to share their special moments of gratitude for her love and say goodbye. There was no mistaking the dull, heavy, rotten, empty, and lonely feeling. It was awful to lose her.

As I watched my siblings—her devoted children—say goodbye to the woman who had birthed us, nurtured us, loved us, respected us, and undeniably represented all that was good in our lives, I could only think of these words—from 1 Corinthians, chapter 13, verse 13: *And now these three remain: faith, hope, and love. But the greatest of these is love.*

I had seen this passage take life in the interaction between Mom and Dad when Dad was passing, and I was seeing it again as we, her children, said goodbye. This woman was a fighter. She was the CEO. She was the wind beneath our wings, and she was not going to let dementia steal her last earthly message to her seven children. She was determined to give us *the greatest gift of love in letting us know that she remembered that we were her children and she was our mom.*

As distance prevented one of my younger brothers from getting to Mom immediately, he phoned. At this point, Mom had not talked in three days. We were monitoring her breathing, listening to the "death gurgle," and dosing her with morphine with the assistance of the hospice staff.

It was Saturday afternoon, and I had just finished positioning a dose of morphine in the left back pocket of her cheek, when my cell phone rang. It was Jamesy.

I held up the phone to her ear as we heard our beautiful brother tell her he loved her and that he and his wife, whom she adored, were healthy and happy, as were his three children. He talked with her for some time about his daughters' activities with Irish step-dancing and A+ grades, and outstanding soccer stories of her grandson. He told her that he and his family loved her dearly—and that it was time for her to go to Dad.

As I held the phone to her ear, the woman who had not spoken in days surged through dementia's stronghold and resurfaced as our mom. "I love you, Jamesy," she said. She was his mom, and she let him know that she *remembered* her role in his life. I held her weakened body in my arms, and thanked her for the moment of joy she had just given all of us, especially Jamesy. Those were her last words. "I love you, Jamesy," words spoken from her memory, a memory that was safely stored within her soul.

Scoreboard: Mom and her seven children, 1; Dementia, 0

Take that, Dementia.

Two days later, our hospice nurse told us that it was likely that Mom would die within twenty-four hours. They were surprised that she had lasted as long as she had. They thought she would have died over the weekend, yet it was Tuesday and she was still alive. I was so grateful that she was holding on. She still needed to see Tom, who couldn't get to Mom any sooner than Wednesday morning. He was doing everything he could to get there.

"Please, tell her I'm coming. Please. Please, tell her." He pleaded through his messages.

By now, Mom had no kidney function, blue feet, gurgling breath, and a very stiff body. It was against all medical science that she would still be alive on Wednesday morning. In fact, when the hospice team said goodbye that night, they told us it had been an honor to get to know our sweet mom. They left, knowing that through the night I would be *doing what had to be done*—administering the morphine in her left back cheek pocket to lessen the immense pain of dying.

On Wednesday morning at 10:00 a.m., our hospice nurse and chaplain returned again to Mom's room expressing their complete shock that she was still alive.

"Is there anyone or anything that she may be waiting for? Did she get a chance to say goodbye to all of you?" The chaplain asked.

I showed them my brother's text message. He was the only one left of all of us whose "goodbye" she had not heard. I suddenly got it. I understood why Mom was desperately hanging on to her life. Just like she had proven to us in her last words to Jamesy, she was proving to us again that *her memory of being a mom was still in the memory of her maternal soul.*

When we were children, Mom would wait in bed "with one eye open" until we got home at night, needing to know that those she loved and protected were safe. She couldn't sleep until she heard the sound of us coming up the staircase. This maternal safeguard was still alive in her as she fought to stay alive and hear my brother's voice—as she had waited to hear all of our voices. She wasn't about to enter perpetual sleep until she knew firsthand that we were all OK.

At 11:00 a.m., my youngest brother, as promised, walked into Mom's room and assured her that he was well and that his wife and his children were healthy, happy, and thriving. He told her it was time for her to be with Dad. His large, Irish, broad-shouldered body appeared dwarfed, as he, her youngest son, left the room blinded by tears. By then, it was 4:00 p.m.

After Tom left, I administered another dose of morphine and then lay down next to Mom in her bed. It was just the two of us. "I love you, Mom," I told her, but she didn't move.

Three hours after Tom left I heard her whisper, "Margaret." I lifted my head from her chest and felt shivers go down my spine. *Thank you, God. Thank you for letting me hear the sound of the sisters' reuniting souls.*

As she took her last breath, I held her tiny head close to my breasts, my arms wrapped around her like a bunting blanket and my shoulders strapped over her in protection. My own heart stopped with her last breath. I slowly released my grip from her frail lifeless body. With my fingers still on the small of her back, where they no longer felt her lungs working, my toes tingled. When I looked down at my feet, I saw that I was wearing Mom's little lace ankle socks. I smiled and knew I would be OK. *You tried to take her earlier. You tried to take away her biggest accomplishment in life. You tried to take away her motherhood, and you lost.* Goodbye, Dementia.

Mom died October 31st—the eve of All Saints' Day, one of the holiest times of the year in the Roman Catholic faith to pass into heaven. She died peacefully in the same solid oak bed that was part of the "can't live without" items that my Dad had brought with him in his move to assisted living, the same bed she'd shared with my dad for 59 years. Over her bed were the portraits of her seven children.

As I lay there with her lifeless body, an overwhelming sense of what we had shared drifted through my mind as I replayed the last several years of seeking to learn, seeking to protect, and ultimately seeking to care more about whom she was than ever before in my 52 years. I had received a remarkable spiritual and life lesson after healing, caring, loving, crying, and praying with both Mom and Dad. It became crystal clear. The lesson I had learned lay in the center of Mom's happiness.

She had been loved.

> **"**And now these three remain: faith, hope, and love. But the greatest of these is love."
>
> *1 Corinthians 13:13*

Mom is buried on Dad's left side, the side where she sat for breakfast all of their years of marriage. The side where Dad would place his poetic napkin far enough away from her coffee and her bagel so that marmalade would not spill on his poetry.

She is buried wearing an Irish scarf and holding a morning napkin.

Now it is my turn.

Manny + Marshal

Roses are Red
Violets are Blue
Who could I ever love
More than I love you?
No one is the answer,
For sure that is true!
Remember...
I will NEVER FORGET
How much I love you!
All my love to you both and of course
that "wonderful Dad" too!
Love,
Mom

Never forget this.